From Challenge to
CHAMPION

From Challenge to
CHAMPION

10 Factors That Can Drastically Improve
Your Child's Challenging Behavior

MILDRED CARSON

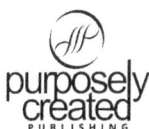

purposely
created
PUBLISHING

FROM CHALLENGE TO CHAMPION
Published by Purposely Created Publishing Group™
Copyright © 2019 Mildred Carson

All rights reserved.

Printed in the United States of America

ISBN: 978-1-64484-049-8

Special discounts are available on bulk quantity purchases by book clubs, associations and special interest groups.
For details email: sales@publishyourgift.com or call (888) 949-6228.
For information log on to: www.PublishYourGift.com

First and foremost, I would like to thank my heavenly Father for His favor, grace, and mercy. I dedicate this book to my parents, Edward and Valarie J. Carson, my grandparents, Julious and Frances Hart, and to my siblings, Adriane Carson-Johnson and Everett Carson. Thank you for always loving and supporting me through this extraordinary journey called life. Special acknowledgement to my two handsome, intelligent nephews that are more like my sons, Jaylon and Landon Carson. God truly blessed me when he chose you to be my family. Thank you for your dedication and endless love and support.

TABLE OF CONTENTS

MY STORY

I am Dr. Mildred, a compassionate, bubbly, board-certified pediatrician, children's behavioral coach, author, speaker and children's health advocate. I have proudly served on multiple child advocacy boards, held several academic and administrative appointments, and am an active member of Delta Sigma Theta Sorority, Inc. I have over 15 years in clinical practice and currently serve as medical director of a behavioral health agency. This has allowed me to see over 10,000 kids with 10,000 personalities and has given me over 10,000 opportunities to make a difference. Helping children to be happy and healthy is my goal, but a significant amount of my practice has been committed to counseling and providing effective plans for implementing more structure for children with behavioral issues.

I have always loved learning and have excelled. Graduating Summa Cum Laude from college, being accepted to several medical schools with multiple scholarships and successfully finishing pediatric residency were some of the highlights of my academic career. I love what I do, but it didn't start out so smoothly. At the age of 3, I vividly remember being excited to start school early and ride the bus like a big girl. It's funny what stands out as you reflect on your childhood—in my case, it is the memory of being the smallest one on the bus, requiring help from my bus driver, Nathan, to assist me with getting on and off every morning and afternoon. Over the course of those bus rides, the once bright, enthusiastic, interactive child began to withdraw from classroom interactions. Initially, my teacher eagerly answered questions, however, perhaps I asked more questions and/or took up more classroom time than the teacher liked and as a result she no longer called on me to answer questions or help with classroom activities. It was my teacher's aide, Ms. Brailey, who was the first to notice the dimming of the light of the bright-eyed, happy little girl. At the first parent-teacher conference, Ms. Brailey informed my parents that I was being ignored and neglected by my teacher. Ms. Brailey, my advocate, gave me and my family the insight necessary to make sure I had the chance to become successful. This early childhood experience may seem insignificant, but this type of interaction can change a child's direction. Regardless of age, clear communication is key to success in all aspects of life. I recognize from my own experience that children internalize negativity and that it can be reflected in their behavior. In my case, my interest in classroom participation diminished.

I am passionate about building better behaviors and better families by helping parents understand and advocate for their child, know their personality, increase communication, decrease stress, create structure, gain control and effectively discipline. My coaching program was created to help kids reach their full potential and through it, I look forward to helping the next 10,000 kids, 10,000 personalities and 10,000 families. If you are ready to get your child on the right track, join countless other parents and become a #ChampMom and #ChampDad today. **WATCH YOUR CHILD TRANSFORM FROM CHALLENGE TO CHAMPION.**

INTRODUCTION

First, let me begin by thanking you for trusting me to be your partner as we embark on our journey to transform your child from challenge to champion. This journey is not going to be easy, but with patience, love, and consistency this book is sure to help produce positive outcomes for you and your child. In drafting this book, I reflected on 15 years of clinical experience of strategies that worked and didn't work, what tools were successful, which were not, and what tips would be most valuable to you the reader. Along the way, I encountered families with various difficulties, challenges, and obstacles with behavior, so rest assured you are not alone. In the following pages you will not find a quick fix, a magic pill, or a Disney-like ending, but you will find sound, sensible advice and tools based on real life experience to better equip you for the road ahead. Now, sit back, relax, take a deep breath and watch the positive changes unfold. I wish you all my very best!

WHO AM I?

Behaviors Are Affected by Personality

How children respond to discipline is largely connected to the type of personality they have. Knowing your children's personality type will give insight on the best approach to communicating with your children and how to structure discipline and give them what they need to prosper. Although personality can be a complicated subject, this section provides a simplified way to view personality types. For the purpose of this book, we will be discussing the following personality types: easy, shy, spirited, fearless and outgoing. Although children can display characteristics from multiple types, they usually have a dominant primary personality. Regardless of your child's personality type, ensure that your child feels like a champion daily.

EASY

These are the kids that are cheerful and don't anger easily. They usually don't mind new places, people, environments, or situations. Easy kids can become lost in the crowd because they don't require as much time and attention. These kids usually don't ask for much and are often the peacemakers and concede to their siblings. They are so easy that sometimes they don't get as much praise as they should because they are constant in their positivity. Don't neglect their need for attention, whether they seem to require it or not, because they can become lonely and depressed.

Quick Tip: Be sure to be present. Ask these kids about their day, upcoming events and activities. Be mindful and don't let the accomplishments of the other children overshadow the easy child's achievements.

SHY

Shy kids resist change and need time to transition between activities. These children are gentle and soft-hearted. They have issues with rejection and shouldn't be rushed into things. They may require extra time for decision making and can be sensitive to external stimuli. The shy child craves stability and extra support.

Quick Tip: Gently encourage these children to step outside of their comfort zone and try things, such as new foods, playing a musical instrument, taking an acting or drama class or even public speaking.

SPIRITED

Spirited kids are often very active and impulsive. They tend to be impatient, very intense, rigid, and are known to be moody, having many daily highs and lows. These strong-willed children need structure and parents have to focus on not getting frustrated and staying calm. Clear directions are required and they can benefit from burning off extra energy.

Quick Tip: Avoid power struggles by establishing a routine and sticking to it, using their strengths as a foundation.

FEARLESS

Fearless children are very confident from an early age. They enjoy independence and autonomy. Do not allow them to become bored. They can find themselves in dangerous situations fairly quickly. These children are explorers and are always into something. Keep their minds stimulated and their bodies moving to decrease the risk of injury.

Quick Tip: Keep these kids physically active and entertained.

OUTGOING

Outgoing children are very friendly and personable. They have bubbly personalities, are excellent conversationalists, and are fun to be around. Allow these kids to be involved in extracurricular activities to foster their social skills. These children tend to be talkative and need opportunities to express themselves.

Quick Tip: These kids tend to be very successful with unstructured activities but can find challenges in structured environments. They also have difficulty understanding kids with another personality type and why they are different. This is a great opportunity to teach acceptance of others, to help them realize that our differences are what make us unique, and to demonstrate that different personalities and interests make the world a more interesting place to live.

Things to Remember

Things to Remember

Things to Remember

Things to Remember

2

WHAT IS YOUR STYLE?

Parenting Techniques

Parenting style is defined as a psychological construct representing standard strategies that parents use in their child rearing. Diane Baumrind created a categorization of parenting styles in the US in the 1960s. Dr. Baumrind was a clinical and developmental psychologist known for her research on how parents and children relate in the home. The three Baumrind parenting styles are authoritarian, authoritative, and permissive. A forth style, uninvolved, was later added by psychologists Maccoby and Martin. They differ by discipline style, nurturance, expectations and communication. A child's temperament/personality should be considered and a combination of parenting styles are often necessary during different situations and periods of a child's life.

AUTHORITARIAN (DISCPLINARIAN)

Based on Baumrind's observations, these parents are controlling, set very high expectations, and are demanding without offering warmth. The discipline is usually harsh and the child has little control. The products of this parenting style are children who have difficulty completing tasks and are unsure of themselves. These children may be socially withdrawn and have difficulty forming trusting relationships.

AUTHORITATIVE (JUST RIGHT)

These parents set high expectations but are warm and responsive to their child's needs. Authoritative parents listen and give advice, and unlike authoritarian parents they are flexible, not rigid. Authoritative parents use reason, explain rules, and use warm communication. The children raised with this style tend to be independent, popular, and have high self-esteem. Baumrind states that this style has the most positive outcomes as demonstrated by academically strong and emotionally stable children.

PERMISSIVE (INDULGENT)

Permissive parents are very warm but do not set any limits. These kids are allowed to do as they please and may grow up not understanding that society will impose limits. Parents under this umbrella do not give direction; they let children decide for themselves, thus they have difficulty functioning within society's limits. Baumrind notes that the effect on children may be that they do not have self-control, are impulsive, and have difficulty adapting to adult life.

UNINVOLVED

Uninvolved parents do not use any particular style of discipline. Often, the children do what they want because the parent either does not care or does not have the appropriate information. There are no expectations set for the child, little nurturing, and communication is limited.

Things to Remember

_____

_____

_____

_____

_____

_____

_____

_____

_____

_____

_____

_____

_____

_____

_____

_____

Things to Remember

Things to Remember

_____

_____

_____

_____

_____

_____

_____

_____

_____

_____

_____

_____

_____

_____

_____

_____

Things to Remember

3

DIET MATTERS
Adjust Dietary Components

I'm sure you have all heard the old phrase, "You are what you eat." Believe it or not, there is some truth to this. Proper nutrition is important to appropriate brain and bodily functions. Many foods today have lots of added sugar, caffeine, dyes, and preservatives. These additions can negatively affect behaviors in those with a predisposition for hyperactivity and mood disturbances. Decreasing additive exposure can drastically reduce unwanted behaviors in children.

SUGAR

Avoid extra and added sugars in foods and beverages. Sugar can increase activity in kids that already have hyperactive tendencies. The rapid ups and downs in blood sugar can cause irritability and grumpiness. The drops in blood sugar can trigger cravings for more sweets and it becomes a vicious cycle. Also remember that insulin, the hormone that is released to keep blood sugar levels from getting too high, has to work overtime, possibly increasing your child's risk for diabetes.

The juices that are favorites of toddlers and young children usually contain a lot of added sugar. Try to choose no sugar added natural juices or lightly flavored water instead. Limit the amount of juice allowed in your child's daily diet. When juice is first introduced, dilute it with water so your child will never know the difference. Remember also that water is a very important beverage for proper bodily function. After the age of 1, a child can have water freely. Do not introduce candy to your child for the first 2 years of life and then allow it sparingly. Do not forget that sugar is addictive. Help your child by avoiding it when you can. Habits formed as children often follow us into adulthood.

JUNK FOOD

Kids who eat fast food on a regular basis are taking in added sugar, preservatives, dyes, and chemicals. All of these additives can cause severe behavioral changes in children. This diet is low in nutrition, high in fat and cholesterol, and sets children up for chronic disease. The rates of obesity and diabetes in children are at an all-time high. Try to feed your child cleaner, healthier foods. Use fresh or fresh frozen instead of canned foods, increase fruits and vegetables, limit portion sizes, choose healthier snacks, and add water to your child's diet. Prepare as many meals at home as you can so you know what your child is eating. Fast food should be a treat, not a regular source of nutrition. Avoid processed foods like sandwich meats, noodles, and microwaveable foods.

FOOD COLORING AND DYE

Red dyes in foods and beverages have been shown to increase hyperactive behaviors. Reading labels is important to identify products containing red dyes. Products you may never expect could have large amounts of these chemicals. Just because a product is not red does not mean it is free of red coloring or dyes. Be diligent and do your research.

CAFFEINE

Caffeine is a stimulant that people use to increase alertness and decrease drowsiness. The most common caffeine containing products are chocolate, coffee, tea, energy drinks, and soft drinks/sodas. Energy drinks are especially dangerous, not only for children, but also adults due to fatal disturbances in the normal heart rhythm. These drinks not only contain caffeine, but also include other ingredients that are not healthy for children. Caffeine can hinder sleep and cause anxiety. Conversely, caffeine withdrawal can trigger nervousness, headaches, and irritability. Avoid caffeine in your child's diet due to its addictive nature. The use of caffeine in children can cause palpitations, tremors, and sleep disturbances.

FOOD ALLERGY, SENSITIVITY OR INTOLERANCE

Issues with food allergies, sensitivities, or intolerances can cause children to display abnormal behaviors. Reactions to food can cause inflammation in the brain and lead to meltdowns, irritability, depression and anxiety. There has been extensive research showing a link between brain inflammation and mood disorders, autism, depression, and anxiety. Food allergies in children can cause respiratory infections, gastrointestinal symptoms and hyperactive symptoms that mimic attention deficit hyperactivity disorder (ADHD). The most common allergens are dairy, nuts, eggs and soy. Children with true food allergies require complete avoidance of those foods and sometimes special meal preparations. The limitations on diet can significantly affect family socialization and planned activities. The extra preparations and planning can increase parental stress, however, simple substitutions can make life easier for parents and food choices more palatable for children. For example, soy milk can be substituted for cow's milk. Consider seeking parental support groups and browse blogs to obtain advice and recommendations regarding your child's specific allergies. Healthcare providers are an invaluable resource for information and referrals to dieticians and nutritionists. All caretakers must be aware of allergies and if prescribed, have proper training in the use of an EpiPen. Severe food allergies can cause respiratory distress and even death.

PRESERVATIVES

There are several preservatives that can cause behavioral problems in children. MSG, a common additive used for flavor enhancement, can cause mood changes. Similarly, sodium benzoate is commonly used in juice products marketed to kids and in studies was found to cause hyperactive behaviors. Nitrates and nitrites, often found in sandwich meats, can cause an increase in mania, and abnormal mood state. Keeping a thorough food diary is helpful whenever alterations in behavior are suspected to be caused by food or food additives.

Things to Remember

Things to Remember

Things to Remember

Things to Remember

4

REST EASY

Learn the Importance of Sleep

Children require adequate sleep to function at their best. Adequate amounts of sleep vary by age.

- Newborns from age 0 to 3 months require 14 to 17 hours

- Infants from age 4 to 11 months require 12 to 15 hours

- Toddlers from age 1 to 2 years require 11 to 14 hours

- Preschoolers from age 3 to 5 years require 10 to 13 hours

- School Aged from age 6 to 13 years require 9 to 11 hours

- Teens from age 14 to 17 years require 8 to 10 hours

Not getting enough sleep during early childhood has been linked to cognitive and behavioral problems later in life. Lack of sleep as a child can cause sleep disturbance issues well into adolescence and adulthood. Children that do not get enough sleep are moody, have more frequent meltdowns, temper tantrums, do not perform or learn as well as they should in school, tend to fall asleep during the day and are hard to get up in the morning,

The brain and the body need time to rest. Our body repairs itself during sleep. If children do not get proper rest, their bodies are not repairing daily damage, which can lead to disease later in life. Don't forget that habits we develop as children often follow us into adulthood. Good sleeping habits are no exception, so let's start them early getting enough and proper sleep.

QUALITY OF SLEEP

Children not only need adequate amounts of sleep, they also need good quality sleep. Inadequate rest increases the risk of children being anxious, hyperactive, having poor attention spans and becoming more impulsive. Difficulty falling asleep or staying asleep can also be caused by other medical issues like Obstructive Sleep Apnea, anxiety, and breathing issues. Assess how hard it is to awaken your child in the mornings. If he has excessive drowsiness during the day and moodiness is worse than expected, seek assistance from your child's provider.

NAPS

Naps are important for young children, as daytime sleep is usually required for kids to get enough rest. The duration of naps depends on the age of your child. Kids between the ages of 6 and 12 months usually require two naps a day, lasting from 20 minutes to several hours. Toddlers between the ages of 1 and 3 usually need an afternoon nap lasting 1-3 hours to fulfill the daily sleep requirement of about 14 hours. Pre-schoolers aged 3-5 still take afternoon naps in addition to their 11-12 hour nightly sleep average. Naps after the age of 5 are not as common due to the decreased overall daily sleep average of 10-11 hours. Naps allow your child to recharge and refresh. We all know how fussy and whiny kids are when they are tired, so allow proper time for naps. Be sure not to allow napping too late in the afternoon or for longer than 3 hours to avoid affecting night time restfulness. Short power naps of 20-30 min can be very effective as a quick refresher to improve mood and alertness in older children and adolescents as well.

SLEEP HYGIENE

Proper sleep hygiene can help children obtain a good night's rest. Children should have a consistent bedtime so they will know what time they're expected to go to bed every night. They should also have a structured bedtime routine that allows time to wind down. This should include a bath, a story and/or prayer. The bedroom is for sleep and it should be associated with sleep, not playtime, TV time, or entertainment time.

Allow children to fall asleep independently of you so they can develop self-soothing skills. Remove electronic devices from the room at bedtime to decrease stimulation. Not having a television in your child's bedroom reinforces that the bedroom is for sleep time, not for entertainment time.

Many parents still have kids sleeping with them and this is not recommended due to safety concerns. Children should never sleep with you, even as infants. Sudden infant death syndrome (SIDS) is a common cause of death in children under a year of age. There have also been numerous cases of death due to a parent rolling onto their infant during the night. If you currently have your infant or child sleeping in your bed, I strongly suggest discontinuing this practice immediately. Place children in their own beds and lay with them until they fall asleep. Use a reward system to encourage them to continue sleeping in their own bed. Do not be surprised if you wake up and your child is in your bed. It will take time to break this habit and much patience is required. I suggest that new parents place a bassinet next to the bed, a crib in the room, or a co-sleeper bed.

SLEEP SOLUTIONS

Many kids with developmental and behavioral delays or difficulties have issues with sleep. There are over the counter (OTC) medications and prescription options available to help improve sleep. Never give your child sleeping medications without consulting his/her provider. Some kids may need to have naps eliminated to allow a decent bedtime. Noise reduction can be of benefit to children as well, providing a decrease in stimulation, while others may need soft music to aid in falling asleep. Have a cut off time for electronic devices used at night.

Sleep can also be affected by nightmares and night terrors. Nightmares are frightening dreams during REM (rapid eye movement) sleep that are considered normal and are a regular stage of development. The exact cause of nightmares is unknown, however, they can be precipitated by medications, experiences, and scary movies or shows. Be sure to filter what children watch online, what they watch on television, and the video games they play. Other nightly sleep disruptions from which your child might suffer are night terrors, which are usually recurrent, frequent episodes of fear during deep non-REM sleep that can include sweating, flailing, screaming, kicking, crying and even sleep walking. They usually occur a few hours after a child falls asleep and are the product of partial waking from sleep. Night terrors can occur at any age but are very common between 2 and 6 years of age. They are noted more commonly in kids that are overly tired, ill, stressed, exposed to too much caffeine, starting a new medication, or are in a new environment. Parents are very disturbed by night terrors because the children seem awake but often don't recognize them and are afraid and inconsolable. They tend to happen around the same time of night and can be helped by awakening the child prior to the episodes.

Nocturnal enuresis or bedwetting is another issue kids face at night. It is defined as the loss of bladder control at night. Bedwetting is normal up until the age of 7 when children should gain nighttime bladder control. There is a small percentage of children that will still wet the bed at night after age 7, and this is considered normal. Often in these cases, there is a strong family history of bedwetting, usually by one or both parents. Risk factors for bed wetting include being male, having a family history of nocturnal enuresis, attention deficit hyperactivity disorder (ADHD), stress and anxiety. Complications of nighttime wetting are rashes, embarrassment, and lack of confidence to attend sleep overs and/or camps. Do not punish children for bedwetting and let them know it is not their fault. Remind them that many other kids have the same issue. Some factors that contribute to nocturnal enuresis include:

- A small bladder - a bladder that has not developed enough to hold the urine produced at night.

- Chronic constipation - urine and stool elimination are controlled by the same muscles, which can sometimes stop functioning properly.

- Urinary tract infections (UTIs) - infection may make it impossible for children to control their urination.

- Diabetes – wetting at night when previously dry can be an early sign of diabetes.

▶ Sleep apnea- bedwetting can be a sign of obstructive sleep apnea (interrupted breathing during sleep).

▶ Urinary tract or nervous system issues - a congenital problem of either system can be cause bedwetting.

▶ Lack of recognition of a full bladder - immature nerves that control the bladder especially during deep sleep.

▶ A deep sleeper - some children sleep very deeply and are not even aware they have wet the bed until the next morning.

▶ Hormonal issues - improper production of anti-diuretic hormone (ADH), the hormone that slows urine production at night.

▶ Sexual abuse - abuse should be considered in a child who was dry at night for an extended time and who began bedwetting again. There will likely be other signs including chronic UTIs, vaginal pain and genital discharge.

Bedwetting usually resolves on its own, but in some cases may indicate a medical problem. Consult your child's provider if a child that has been dry for months starts wetting again, and the wetting is accompanied by painful urination, unusually colored urine, hard stools, snoring or increased thirst. The treatment of nocturnal enuresis not caused by a medical condition usually requires changes in habits or supportive therapy. These include setting cut off times for beverages at night, making the child urinate immediately before bed, awakening the child to use the restroom in the middle of the night, bedwetting alarms and giving rewards for dry nights. I recommend the use of waterproof mattress covers, disposable mattress pads, and Pull-Ups during the time of transition to dry nights. Bed wetting alarms are an option to discourage bed wetting and there are several different types of alarms that awaken the child when wetness is detected.

For children who have been abused or have had any type of life trauma, seek counseling or therapy to help them to deal with the underlying issue to improve the wetting. There are medications that can be prescribed to help decrease nighttime wetting through decreasing urine production and calming the bladder. These medications include desmopressin, oxybutynin, hyoscyamine and imipramine. Medications may or may not be prescribed to your child based on the treatment plan determined by his or her provider.

Sleep plays a vital role in our physical health. Setting healthy habits around sleep sets the framework for your child's success. Many of these issues are related to normal childhood development and are often self-limited. Monitor for problems and know there are sleep solutions available.

Things to Remember

_____

_____

_____

_____

_____

_____

_____

_____

_____

_____

_____

_____

_____

_____

_____

_____

Things to Remember

_____

_____

_____

_____

_____

_____

_____

_____

_____

_____

_____

_____

_____

_____

_____

_____

Things to Remember

_____

_____

_____

_____

_____

_____

_____

_____

_____

_____

_____

_____

_____

_____

_____

_____

Things to Remember

5

LET'S LIMIT THE MEDIA

Don't Let Media Hijack Their Minds

The term media refers to the means or channels of general communication. There are many different types of available media in this technological society we live in. Cell phones are so available and abundant that many kids have their own. When setting daily media time limits remember that television, tablets, cell phones, games, computers and iPads are all included. You as the parent control the home screen time, but don't forget that most schools require some computer use for school work and homework, and that time is also included.

LIMITS

Children spend multiple hours a day on media outlets. The use of media in schools has contributed to the increase in daily exposure. Too much media time can decrease the amount of time kids have to sleep, talk, play, and study. Know what your children are watching and limit the screen time. Designate times and locations to be media free. Do not allow cell phones at the dinner table. Social interaction has drastically decreased in our children due to electronic devices. Overuse of electronics can cause social isolation, which can lead to depression and anxiety.

SOCIAL MEDIA

Social media sites like Facebook, Instagram, Snapchat, and Pinterest are very popular among children of varied ages. The accessibility of the Internet has made bullying, depression, childhood/adolescent stress and anxiety more prominent. Once something is on the Internet it is almost impossible to remove, making negative situations linger longer. Keep an eye on your children's pages on social media to help protect them from predators and scammers. Social media can be dangerous, so do not take it lightly. Teach your children not to give out any information online, including where they live, where they attend school, or where they work. Remind your children to never send private pictures of themselves through texts, emails, or online. MONITOR YOUR CHILDREN!

APPROPRIATE MEDIA

Media should be approached with a plan and tailored based on the age of your child. Not all media is appropriate for all children. You must be selective about your child's media exposure. Emails are required for registration on many sites and that is because only those over the age of 16 are meant to have an email address. This age limit was purposefully used to limit children's access to certain websites, but it has not been very effective.

Small children under 18 months of age should be shielded from media with limited screen time. The developing brain can be negatively impacted by media and can contribute to hyperactivity, attention issues, and delays.

MEDIA RESOURCES

Due to increasing risk to children and thus society, the American Academy of Pediatrics released recommendations to help parents navigate media. Media can be used in positive and constructive ways for learning, but negative influence is also possible. There are several resources to help the media maze. Develop a plan to limit exposure time and be consistent.

Things to Remember

Things to Remember

Things to Remember

Things to Remember

6

KEEP IT MOVING!

Activity Is Good for the Body and the Brain

Physical activity plays a vital role in physical, mental, and emotional health. Exercise provides a release for excess energy. Play can be therapeutic for children and offers improvements in socialization skills. Some sports are more beneficial to some kids than to others.

EXERCISE

Exercise is great for the mind, body, and spirit. We need to add daily exercise to children's schedules to help combat the childhood obesity epidemic. Exercise will help your child burn off some of his/her excessive energy. Physical activity can aid in improved sleep for children. Exercising also releases endorphins (feel good hormones) that can trigger happy feelings and decrease mood swings.

LEARNING TO PLAY

Play can be therapeutic to children with behavioral issues. It can help to improve attention and social skills. Set daily play times and make them short for children with short attention spans. Encourage fantasy play and have children express their feelings through characters. Classic games can be adapted by increasing challenges as your child develops skills. Choose games that help them to increase attention and memory, understand consequences, problem solve and develop organizational skills.

Playtime raises the levels of neurotransmitters that improve attention. Sports participation allows a child to work on self-esteem and build social skills. Choose sports that are more structured, provide small group or one-on-one interactions, and allow the practice of self-control. Kids with behavioral issues benefit from sports that allow safe physical contact and that infrequently requires direct competition with others. Always communicate special needs with coaches. Some modifications may be needed to help your child be as successful as possible.

NOT CREATED EQUAL

Not all activities are created equal. You want to keep your child stimulated mentally and physically, however, avoid using media to entertain your child. Some cartoons actually teach usable information, but many don't. Do not let television, tablets, cell phones, or video games babysit or raise your child; you **will not** like the results. Instead, play board games that will help them with memory, attention, and concentration. Get out in the yard and play kickball, or simply have a fun dance-off.

GAMES ARE US

Choose games and activities for kids that will help with self-regulation, memory building, and improving attention. There are options to use instead of media to keep kids entertained. Here are some examples of recommended games and activities: Simon Says, Chinese Checkers, I Spy, Chutes and Ladders, Clue, Red Light/Green Light, and Hide and Seek. Board games give the eyes and brain a break from electronic devices.

Things to Remember

_____

_____

_____

_____

_____

_____

_____

_____

_____

_____

_____

_____

_____

_____

_____

_____

Things to Remember

Things to Remember

Things to Remember

7

BE POSITIVE

Positive Reinforcement Is Better than the Negative Alternative

Children respond more favorably to positive words and actions than to negative talk and interactions. Positivity helps children build self-esteem, display confidence and develop self-motivational skills. Parents should be generous with praise and keep criticism constructive to avoid self-doubt and insecurity.

REWARD ME

Small rewards when your child accomplishes a goal can be super helpful and encouraging. Everyone likes receiving gifts; I know I do! These small tokens can help boost your child's self-esteem, which also builds confidence. Improved confidence translates into less negative behavior. You can use stickers, hand stamps, and small prizes in addition to your words as rewards.

PRAISE ME

Being praised helps children to be more motivated. Motivated kids feel pride in the things they do. Subsequently, they try harder and stick to activities longer. Praise your children for completing activities and acknowledge the effort even if they don't. Do not compare a child to other children, even if you are trying to compliment her. Compare the child's improvement to her previous attempt. Try, however, not to interrupt kids who are focusing to praise them so that you do not throw them off task.

BE ENCOURAGED

We all need to hear a positive word from others sometimes. Prompt your child to continue positive behaviors through encouragement. Encourage your child to try new situations, foods, and activities. If children encounter difficulties, show them your support through solving the problem together. Do not tell children they have done a good job when they have not put forth effort. Encourage them to do better. They know when you are not being honest. Try not to pressure your kids into improvement. Instead, encourage them to perform to the best of their ability.

ATTENTION PLEASE

Children that misbehave often get more attention than those that don't. Let's change the way we approach these situations and praise the children who are doing as they are told with hopes that the misbehaving child will notice the praise. Remember that any attention, even bad attention, is still attention. Acknowledging it will only encourage the continuation. Ignore the negative behaviors as much as possible, but always correct dangerous behaviors immediately.

AFFIRMATIONS

Speak it into existence! Start speaking positivity over your kids before they can talk or walk and don't stop. Even when they are infants, talk to them and tell them all the great things they are and all the things you want for their life. Use general terms like you are kind, you are unique, and you are special. If they hear it at home first, they will believe it and they can achieve it. Do not let the negative world have them believe they are inferior, not beautiful, or not worthy.

ENVIRONMENT

Your children's environment has a large impact on them as they grow and mature. Be very mindful of who your child is exposed to and limit negative influences as much as possible. Anyone who treats your children badly or exposes them to inappropriate language and behaviors needs to be eliminated. We can't always help where we live, but do your best to decrease your child's exposure to drugs, sex, and crime. Monitor what they watch on TV, their Internet use, and the games they own and play. Know your child's friends and be very particular about sleep overs and what outside persons are allowed around your child.

Things to Remember

Things to Remember

Things to Remember

Things to Remember

8

DISCIPLINE ME

Guide Me Please

Discipline is the practice of training people to obey rules or a code of behavior, using punishment to correct disobedience. Most people think discipline means spanking a child, but that is not always the correct solution. Discipline can also consist of time out, taking away toys/activities/games, ignoring unwanted behaviors, and discussions. Age, development, temperament and personality should be considered when deciding on discipline techniques. Remember that adjustments or modifications may be needed for developmentally challenged or sensory altered children. All children need structure and rules to obey. Children are born with an empty slate and it is up to us to teach them right from wrong. They are trying to figure it out as they go and adults set the foundation of right and wrong by what we do and don't allow.

TYPE ME

All children are different in how they respond to certain forms of discipline. The type of discipline used should be tailored to the personality type and temperament of your child. Time-out works for some kids while others may only respond to taking away their favorite toy. This is the reason you should know your child's personality type so that you can provide effective discipline. Varying forms of parenting may be required for different situations. Be sure the punishment or consequence fits the action or offense.

BE CONSISTENT

Consistency is the key to continued positive behaviors. Whenever you tell your child that there is going to be a certain consequence for an action, you need to make sure that you are willing to follow through with that consequence. Kids are betting people. They consider their odds, so if nine out of ten times when you say you're going to do something you do not, they are going to take the chance. If you normally do what you say you're going to do, then that displays consistency and they will be less likely to take the risk because the odds are not in their favor.

Children need discipline in order to know how to function in everyday life and in society. We must set rules, goals, and expectations, and require our children to abide and live by them. Kids need stability and we provide it through consistency. When kids know what is expected of them at all times, they are better able to perform. If we are not dependable as adults, how can we expect them to be?

TANTRUMS BE GONE

Temper tantrums, also known as hissy fits or meltdowns, are emotional outbursts that happen in toddlers and young children and are considered normal. But they can occur in people at any age under extreme stress, mental disability, or immaturity. Tantrums are a very common way in which children express frustration. They can include screaming, crying, head banging, hitting, stubbornness, and a refusal to follow directions. Some common triggers are being told no, not getting their way, not being able to do something by themselves or the birth of a younger sibling. Kids with language and developmental delays become frustrated when others aren't understanding their wants or needs. If your child has issues with speaking, have him evaluated for speech therapy. Ask him to slow down and use his words instead of screaming, yelling, or crying. Concentrate on decreasing your child's frustration to lessen tantrums. Encourage children to express their frustration in a healthier manner and try to control and limit tantrums whenever possible.

Make sure they understand what is not allowed no matter how angry they get. Hitting, biting, yelling and name calling should never be allowed. Instead, ask children to draw a picture or write about what is upsetting them. Let them know it is okay to walk away or take a break and come back to what is frustrating them. I recommend having a tantrum zone where you send them to have their meltdown. Let children know that when they are ready to talk about it like a big boy or girl, they can come out. Keep an eye on them to ensure their safety, but don't let them know you are watching. Make sure your child is safe, but do not give attention to the negative behaviors. Children use tantrums to get attention and get what they want. It doesn't matter if the attention is good or bad as long as it is attention. If you are not giving it any attention, there will be no reason for it to continue or last as long. The best way to decrease them is to ignore them. You will soon see the decrease in the severity and how quickly the tantrums end.

You can use the power of distraction to stop tantrums in their tracks. When children forget what they are falling out about, it will stop. Do not bribe or promise anything, just distract them. You can use a toy or a cartoon or something that makes the child laugh to move her attention to something else.

One of many reasons for tantrums is that small children often want to be bigger than they are and they become aggravated when they are unable to do it or when someone tries to help. Encourage your child to ask for help or to try again more slowly to get it themselves. Allow your child to make minor choices like choosing a banana or an apple in the lunch box to make them feel like a big kid.

Tantrums also occur when children become grumpy because they are tired. Avoid delaying or skipping regular naps to keep moodiness to a minimum. Keep a consistent bedtime so children won't be overly tired during the day. This will slow the number of meltdowns.

Whatever the reason for the tantrum, keep your cool and set some ground rules. Children learn by example, so don't get angry and yell at the child. How can you tell them not to yell or get angry if you are showing them that behavior is acceptable? Keep your composure and stay calm. Getting upset and yelling displays the behaviors you are telling your child are wrong and will only worsen the tantrums.

THE POWER OF NO!

It is okay to introduce the concept of "no" to children at an early age. At 6 months, when children are learning to grab things, begin teaching them that they shouldn't hit. Stop them by grabbing their hands and saying, "No." If you do this consistently, your child will start to understand that no means don't do that. Let's remember that children don't enter the world knowing everything. They don't know right from wrong. We teach them. Discipline is one of the harder parts of being a parent, but it is very necessary. In life we all are faced with no sometimes and we have to be able to accept it and move forward. As adults, we can't go on our job and have a tantrum if we are told no or do not get our way, so we have to teach our children how life works. Discipline teaches children a value system they will use to guide them through life. The system encourages the development of self-control, self-motivation, and better decision making skills. It should be firm but fair. Discipline allows children to become socially and emotionally mature.

Things to Remember

Things to Remember

Things to Remember

Things to Remember

GOT STRUCTURE?

Consistency Is Key!

Structure is the development of an organized plan to shape and mold behavior. Setting expectations and providing a safe and stable environment encourages healthy development and growth. Assigning routines, supplying consistency, and setting limits strengthens the foundation of positive behavior.

ROUTINES, ROUTINES!

Set a daily schedule for your child. Set times for waking and for snacks, meals, homework and bedtime. Children do better in structured environments and it is your job to give them structure and stability. Children with behavioral issues often react positively to being on a schedule. Daily routines allow children to be their best selves.

FAMILY DYNAMICS

Discipline may be impacted by family structures such as a single-parent home, a blended family home, an interracial family home, or a home of extended family. Single-parent homes often have a parent that is working more than one job or long hours to make ends meet and discipline may not be a top priority. Blended families can present a challenge to discipline due to biological and stepparent differences. Interracial families can face challenges due to the different techniques in discipline among cultures, races, and ethnic backgrounds. Extended families in which multiple people have a say in how children are raised can result in many inconsistencies. Decrease inconsistencies by designating certain aspects of discipline to individuals or families having a plan of discipline that everyone follows.

Kids that are between homes can be stressed, trying to remember how they should behave or what is expected from house to house. Consider a child having to abide by two sets of rules. You can imagine that adapting to multiple situations in both environments is difficult. They may be confused and may not always get it right, so let's remember this and cut them a bit of slack. It is best if both parents or guardians are on the same page and there is consistent structure and discipline on both sides. This would make it easier for the parents and better because the child does not have to adapt her behavior as much.

Families need to be on the same page when raising children. If a family is divided, discipline will not be effective because kids will use splitting. Splitting is a way that kids manipulate their parents or caregivers by playing one against another to get what they want. Don't be fooled by children who are overly sweet to get what they want when they have previously shown negative behaviors. I suggest team meetings to make sure everyone is and remains on the same page when it comes to structure and discipline.

STRONG FOUNDATION

Discipline is a core foundation of raising happy, productive children. Parents have to teach children good from bad and right from wrong. Our value system starts to form at a young age and we must foster positive behaviors early. Everything you allow children to do or prevent them from doing teaches them a life lesson. Make those life lessons count.

SPOILING

It is ok to sometimes reward your child for doing extremely well. But do not make the mistake of letting children think they should be rewarded every time they make a good decision. Being productive and well-behaved is expected, not up for negotiation.

In the case of divorce, custodial parents often feel guilty that the non-custodial parent isn't actively involved, and they often allow the child to get away with more than they should. They find themselves overcompensating for the behavior of the absentee parent. Many grandparents are also guilty of over-providing, under-disciplining, and undermining parents. This is detrimental to families. These situations only make it harder for the children throughout their lives. It takes a village to raise children, but the village has to be respectful and keep the rules consistent.

Structure supports the development of security, the ability to master self-control, and the opportunity to make responsible choices. The goal is to provide an environment conducive to foster emotionally balanced, responsible, self-disciplined members of society.

Things to Remember

Things to Remember

Things to Remember

_____

_____

_____

_____

_____

_____

_____

_____

_____

_____

_____

_____

_____

_____

_____

_____

Things to Remember

10

YOU BETTER NOT!

The Rules of the Game

There are rules of parenting that should not be broken. You should always keep your promises. Do not use bribery because it sets a dangerous precedent. Do not be tempted to give into what a child wants just because it is the path of least resistance. Parents need to set clear boundaries at an early age in order to help children understand rules and respect personal space. Demonstrating respect, providing a positive environment, and decreasing negative influences help your child model positive behaviors.

PROMISES, PROMISES!

Do not make promises that you know you can't keep. Children will test you and play the odds. If 9 out of 10 times you say you are going to do something as a consequence for disobedience and you do not follow through, your child will take chances more often than not. Your child has to be able to trust and believe you. Parents set the example and provide a child's sense of stability. Home should be the constant and the standard for how things should be done. If kids don't feel safe and secure at home, how will they cope and manage outside of the home?

BRIBES

Do not use bribery to get your child to do things. It will backfire every time. In order for bribes to continue to work they have to keep increasing in size and/or cost. Children should do what you say because you are the parent, not because you are giving them something. You will set a bad precedent in which children will never do anything you ask without expecting you to give them something in return. Have discussions with children and explain to them why you would like them to do what you ask. It is human nature to be curious and want to know why.

THE GIVE-IN

Parents sometimes just give kids what they want even when they know they should not. Some common reasons for this action are frustration, guilt, tiredness, and even laziness. Do not be fooled. Being a parent is hard and takes lots of work to produce kids that are healthy physically, mentally, and emotionally. Do not give in to inappropriate behaviors and do not let your guilt negatively impact your child. Give your child as much of a fresh start as you can; leave your baggage at the door.

NO HITTING!

Do not allow your child to hit you, especially in the face. If you let them hit you, they will think it is ok to hit others, and it is NOT. From an early age, children should learn to regard authority and not be allowed to disrespect their parent in that manner. Children have to be taught respect, as they are not born knowing what it means. Every person deserves respect, so parents should exercise it with their children and should expect it from them in return.

HEAR NO EVIL

Be careful what you say around your child. Children are truly like little sponges and they absorb everything. Even if they do not act on it or repeat it at that time, they will remember and eventually you will be faced with the correction. Children should love their parents and caregivers and should not be exposed to negative talk from one about another. It does not matter if no child support has been paid or if visits were missed or promises were broken, a child should not know of such adult concerns. Shield them from the cruel world for as long as possible, as much as you can.

Things to Remember

_____

_____

_____

_____

_____

_____

_____

_____

_____

_____

_____

_____

_____

_____

_____

_____

Things to Remember

Things to Remember

Things to Remember

11

DOSE ME!

Medications and Behavior

Medications can be a great adjunct to help treat many conditions and disorders. Behavioral issues can be improved with appropriate medications, but they can also cause unwanted side effects with improper dosages. Medications cannot and should not replace a healthy diet, regular exercise, or proper rest.

OVER-THE-COUNTER (OTC) DANGERS

Medications can have an effect on your child's behavior and overall health. Always read labels for dosages and directions. Over dosages and improper usage can dangerously alter a child's mood, mental status, or physical health. Diphenhydramine (Benadryl), a medicine commonly used for allergies, can cause excessive drowsiness and disturbed coordination. Ibuprofen (Motrin), a very common and well-known anti-fever medication, can cause dizziness and nervousness. There are many known side effects to over-the-counter medications. Be sure to check interactions between OTC and prescription medications. Over-the-counter medications are usually not regulated by the Federal Drug Administration (FDA) and you have to be very careful when choosing them. Different brands have different quantities and qualities of ingredients. Be sure to research and check with your child's provider prior to starting any new medications.

SCRIPT DUTY

There are several prescription medications available to help with attention and behavior. One of the most common and popular types are stimulants. Many myths and misconceptions exist when it comes to ADHD medications. One of the more common misconceptions held by children is that the medication is making them smart. ADHD medications do not increase intelligence. They allow a child to focus and better absorb and process information. Another misconception commonly held by parents is that their children will be in a zombie-like state if they are given medication. For this reason, many parents are against using them. This misconception, however, is the result of the side effects of older medications like Ritalin. The newer medications tend to have fewer side effects and usually do not cause the zombie effect at proper dosages. If children do experience an increase in side effects, it could mean that the dosage is too high. Parents should monitor for signs of excessive weight loss, moodiness, emotional outbursts, unprovoked anger, or sleep difficulty and report them to their child's provider immediately.

VITAMIN HAPPY

Some believe vitamins may help treat or improve attention and behavioral issues. If there is a vitamin deficiency, replacing those vitamins could be helpful. Be cautious of vitamin over dosage because some can be toxic and dangerous. For example, B vitamins in excess can cause nerve damage, headaches, and elevated liver enzymes. Many kids with special behavioral needs are picky eaters by nature and often have a nutritional imbalance. If you suspect your child is deficient in any vitamins and minerals due to poor diet, speak with a provider about replacement options. In general, children over the age of two should have their diet supplemented with an age-appropriate multivitamin. Be cautious of places that charge you for specialized vitamin regimens guaranteed to help your child's ADHD or behavior problems. There are many scams and scammers that prey on parents who desperately want to help their child without using prescription medications.

HERBALS AND NATURALS

Kids with autism, developmental delays, and attention or sensory issues often suffer from sleep disturbances. A deficiency of melatonin may be a factor in some of these cases. Melatonin is produced by the body naturally to aid the body's sleep cycle. It may be recommended by your child's provider as an addition to the management of your child's issue with sleep when given in proper dosages. Remember that too much of anything can be bad and lead to negative consequences for your child's health. Some herbals can have major interactions with prescription medications and should be added with caution.

DOSE 'EM RIGHT

Medications can be a great help for children with behavioral problems. Correct dosages are important to prevent unwanted side effects. Starting off slowly and titrating up is the best way to prevent side effects and it requires patience on the part of parents and caregivers. It is important to remember that more is not always better. Do not increase the dosages of your child's medications without instruction from his/her provider. Let's keep them safe and productive.

There are several classes of medications used for behavioral issues, including stimulants and non-stimulants, anti-depressants, and Atomoxetine. Stimulants are the most commonly used medication in treating attention deficit hyperactivity disorder (ADHD) and are used to stimulate the Central Nervous System (CNS), creating increased attention, alertness, and energy. Common side effects include issues with sleep, headaches, and decreased appetite (weight loss). Stimulants come in short and long acting forms and are available in pills, liquids, and patches.

Non-stimulants are used for children who cannot tolerate stimulants, as adjunct therapy or as sleep aids. Non-stimulants include medications that are also approved for blood pressure control, depression, and affecting levels of the neurotransmitters in the brain. Common side effects include constipation, dry mouth, a decrease in blood pressure, gastrointestinal issues, suicidal thoughts, increased heart rate, headaches, and dizziness.

CHRONIC DISEASE

Children with chronic diseases like asthma, diabetes, sickle cell or cystic fibrosis are often on multiple medications and their behavior can be affected. Some of these medications are known to cause mood changes and even hyperactivity. Monitor changes in children's behavior when they start a new medication and report it to your child's provider immediately. Being different from other children often puts these kids under social stressors and can add anxiety and depression. Remind children that being unique doesn't make them bad or less important than anyone else.

Medications, whether herbal, over-the-counter, or prescription should be approached with caution. Any medication, if used incorrectly, can have negative effects on physical and mental health. Consult your pharmacist or provider before starting any new medications.

Things to Remember

Things to Remember

Things to Remember

Things to Remember

12

COMMON DIAGNOSES AND ASSOCIATED SYMPTOMS

Common Diagnoses that Affect Behavior

Most children and adolescents display undesired behaviors at some point. In fact, such behavior is expected in normal development. Temper tantrums, mild rebellion, and testing boundaries are all examples of normal behavior. When, however, those behaviors disrupt the child's life dynamics, including family, social, and school environment, it may indicate a more serious condition.

ATTENTION DEFICIT HYPERACTIVITY DISORDER (ADHD)

ADHD is defined by the Diagnostic and Statistical Manual of Mental Disorders, fifth edition (**DSM**-V) as a neurodevelopmental disorder affecting both children and adults. It is described as a "persistent" or on-going pattern of inattention and/or hyperactivity-impulsivity that gets in the way of daily life or typical development. There are three different types of ADHD, predominantly inattentive, predominantly hyperactive-impulsive, and combined. Predominantly inattentive children have difficulty with attention and following instructions. They are easily distracted, forgetful, and have issues with organization. Alternately, predominantly hyperactive-impulsive children are very active and talkative. They are known to fidget, interrupt often, and have problems waiting their turn. A person with a combined form has equal symptoms of inattention and hyperactivity-impulsivity.

Managing the environment is the most important aspect of guiding a child with ADD/ADHD. When the environment is conducive to their behavioral needs, they thrive and require less chastising. Environment involves more than just location. It also includes an atmosphere of patience, a calm tone, and a positive attitude. Successful discipline will require several steps. These include an environment with minimal distractions, established routines, concise single-step commands, calmly repeated directions and clear consequences. These children are often in trouble for not listening or following directions, but recognizing this as a challenge for them allows for better management. Set up a room with as few distractions as possible for completing homework to improve attention and focus. Establish routines to decrease the burden of having to process and manage multiple steps. Avoid multi-step instructions and provide single commands to minimize confusion and the annoying forgetfulness these children display. Accept the fact you will still likely need to repeat instructions more than once due to the nature of the disorder. Be sure to have the full attention of your child when you clearly discuss the consequences of actions and/or lack of action.

OPPOSITIONAL DEFIANT DISORDER (ODD)

Oppositional defiant disorder (**ODD**) is defined by the Diagnostic and Statistical Manual of Mental Disorders, fifth edition (**DSM**-V), as a recurring pattern of negative, hostile, disobedient, and defiant behavior in a child or adolescent, lasting for at least six months without serious violation of the basic rights of others. Symptoms of ODD include throwing repeated temper tantrums, blaming others for mistakes, frequent outbursts of anger and resentment, and being spiteful and revenge seeking. They often swear, use obscene language, refuse to comply with requests and rules, and intentionally annoy or upset others. These kids say mean and hateful things when upset and excessively argue with adults, especially those in authority. The cause of ODD is unknown. It is believed that a combination of genetic, biological, and environmental factors contribute to the condition. These children often have low self-esteem and abuse drugs and alcohol later in life.

Set clear rules and well-defined consequences for these children. This disorder is particularly difficult due to the perceived lack of respect these children display. They require therapy early to help them deal with negative thoughts and actions and find more positive ways to cope with frustration. Therapy can also address issues with poor social skills, stress management, and anger control. Praise these children for any compliance with rules, regulations, and authority. Try to limit situations where the child is in direct conflict with any authority figure to minimize their heightened level of stress.

ANXIETY DISORDERS

The Diagnostic and Statistical Manual of Mental Disorders states that anxiety disorders are a group of mental disorders characterized by significant feelings of anxiety and fear. Anxiety is a worry about future events and fear is a reaction to current events. This worry makes it hard to carry out day-to-day activities and responsibilities. These symptoms often cause problems in all aspects of a person's life and may even manifest in physical symptoms.

Some children have generalized anxiety and others are anxious about certain situations or events. A healthy, well-balanced diet, consistent sleep habits, and regular physical activity will decrease overall stress on the mind and body. In general, try to avoid known stressors and use relaxation, breathing, aroma (lavender, chamomile, bergamot), and music therapy to deescalate panic attacks. Reassure these children with safe, calm, trusting environments, concentrate on stress management, and avoid caffeine to lower anxiety symptoms. Consider parent and child support groups and cognitive behavioral therapy to assist the goal of decreased anxiousness. Cognitive behavioral therapy (CBT) is a psychosocial intervention aimed to change unhelpful distortions, improve emotional regulation, and develop coping mechanisms.

DISRUPTIVE MOOD DYSREGULATION DISORDER (DMDD)

Disruptive mood dysregulation disorder is defined by the Diagnostic and Statistical Manual of Mental Disorders, fifth edition (**DSM-V**), as a childhood disorder (ages 6-18) characterized by a pervasively irritable or angry mood and severe temper tantrums. It is a fairly new diagnosis and is classified as a depressive disorder. Symptoms include frequent angry or aggressive outbursts combined with an angry or irritable mood on days when outbursts do not occur. These children can become physically aggressive and throw things.

DMDD is a relatively new diagnosis, therefore, treatment options are still being researched. Parent training, computer-based training, and psychotherapy (treating mental health problems by talking to a mental health provider) are the most current treatments.

AUTISM SPECTRUM DISORDER

Autism spectrum disorder is a broad range of conditions that include challenges with social skills, speech, and repetitive behaviors. A combination of genetic and environmental factors influence the development of autism. It affects 1 in 59 children and can be diagnosed by 18 months, but more commonly between the ages of 2 and 3. To test for the disorder, pediatricians and primary care providers perform a screening test called MCHAT. This screening tool is completed at 18 months and again at 2 years of age to look for possible signs of autism. The form is completed by the parent and asks multiple questions about a child's behavior. Sensory issues are common with this condition. It can also be associated with seizures and sleep and stomach issues. Symptoms include limited to no eye contact, zero or few smiles, lack of facial expressions, no babbling or baby noises, and no pointing or waving. They give no response to their names being called, have a strong preference for being alone, repeat words or phrases, and resist minor change in routines or environment. These kids have unusual reactions to sounds, tastes, textures, light, touch or smells, have repetitive behaviors like rocking, flapping, spinning, or lining things up, and have unusual eating habits. It is not curable but early detection and treatment is crucial. The goal of therapy is to reduce symptoms and support development and learning. Children younger than 3 years of age can enter an early intervention program and children over 3 years of age can obtain services through school. Common therapies are speech therapy, occupational therapy, behavior therapy, family therapy, anger management, sensory processing and social skills training. A few medication classes, including antipsychotics and sleep aids, can sometimes help symptoms. Associated conditions include attention deficit hyperactivity disorder (ADHD), anxiety, depression and obsessive-compulsive disorder.

Children with autism require discipline and structure to thrive. Most of them are capable of understanding and following basic rules. Communication may have to be adapted with the use of cards, sign language or a board. Timeouts will not work for many children but time away from activities they enjoy, like video games or television, can be effective. Keep directions simple and do not punish for behaviors that cannot be avoided, like hand flapping, rocking, or repetitive noises. Establish relationships early by enrolling your child in half-day daycare, school, or head start to build social skills and decrease the likelihood of social anxiety. Start early intervention (play therapy) services as soon as possible to introduce regular social interactions and optimize social integration and function. Learn the sensory (sound, smell, taste, touch, sight) limitations of your child to prevent sensory overload or overwhelm. Try to minimize drastic changes in his/her environment and slowly and strategically introduce new stimuli.

OBSESSIVE-COMPULSIVE DISORDER

Obsessive-compulsive disorder (OCD) is a mental disorder with which people have excessive thoughts that lead them to have repetitive behaviors. They repetitively perform routines and are unable to control the actions or thoughts associated with those routines. Common behaviors include constant hand washing, counting, hoarding, or checking to see if doors are locked. These routines are usually centered on a theme like germs or fear. Some behaviors like excessive hair pulling, nail biting, or skin picking can cause bodily harm. The actions interfere with the activities of daily living. Some people with OCD perform the compulsions because they think it will prevent something bad from happening while others feel like they simply must. The condition can be associated with anxiety, tics, and an increased risk of suicide. Risk factors include stress, child abuse, and in some cases can follow infection. The mainstay of treatment is counseling {cognitive behavioral therapy (CBT)} along with antidepressants. Cognitive behavior therapy is aimed at subjecting the person to what causes the issue while disallowing the repetitive behaviors. Approximately 1–2% of children are affected by OCD. [1] Obsessive–compulsive disorder symptoms tend to develop more frequently in children that are 10–14 years of age, with males displaying symptoms at an earlier age and a more severe level than the females.[2]

Provide reassurance for children with compulsions due to fear. Consider recommending alternative actions to shift focus to something more positive. Find activities and interests that somewhat normalize or allow for a positive expression of the compulsion. Utilize aroma therapy (cypress, lavender, frankincense, sandalwood) to decrease anxiety and promote relaxation, thereby reducing stress.

SENSORY PROCESSING DISORDER

Sensory processing disorder (SPD, also known as sensory integration dysfunction) describes a condition in which multisensory integration is not adequately processed to provide appropriate responses to the demands of the environment. Sensory integration was defined by occupational therapist Anna Jean Ayres in 1972 as "the neurological process that organizes sensation from one's own body and from the environment and makes it possible to use the body effectively within the environment." [4][5] It can manifest as under- or over-sensitivities. These kids can be oversensitive to light, sound, taste and/or touch. They are often uncoordinated, hard to engage, clumsy, and do not like to be touched. They have unusual responses to pain and temperature and don't handle change well. Treatment is available through occupational therapy, which helps them with activities of daily living and to get used to things that usually bother them.

Children with SPD can process pain very differently. A mild touch may be interpreted as painful by one child while another feels nothing at all in response to an act that should cause pain. In the severest of cases, children display what seems like self-harming behaviors when they are actually just trying to feel something. You will have to learn how your child processes stimuli and responds in order to better help her. You will then be aware of over- or under-sensitivity and can strategically alter the environment and educate others about your child's special needs. Physical and occupational therapy can help with sensory integration. Therapies use stimulating and fun activities to push children without over-stimulating them.

EARLY DIAGNOSIS

As with any disease or disorder, early diagnosis is best for all behavioral and sensory disorders. Parents are often in denial about their child's suspected and proven diagnosis. Everyone wants their child to be normal and it's a very emotional time for most people when their child is diagnosed with a behavioral or developmental disorder. But it is important to remember that there are differences between all children, and your child's uniqueness does not make her any less than anyone else's child. Denying it or not accepting what's going on can negatively impact your child's future. The earlier therapies begin, the better the outcome for the child and family.

If you have an older child that developed more quickly or you see a difference between an older child and a younger child and you believe that something's not quite right, there is nothing wrong with going to the pediatrician or primary care doctor's office to ask questions. There is testing that can be performed at certain ages to give us an idea of whether a child is simply having difficulty or actually has a behavioral disorder. Primary care providers can start services while awaiting appointments to see specialists for a formal diagnosis. If everything is normal, there is no harm or foul, but if something is needed, the earlier services are started, the better. If your primary care provider or your pediatrician expresses some concerns about behavioral or sensory issues in your child, please let them make the referrals. Allow the necessary testing to get the correct diagnosis so that the doctor can offer what's best for your child and give her the best chance to succeed and to reach her fullest potential.

Things to Remember

Things to Remember

Things to Remember

Things to Remember

_____

_____

_____

_____

_____

_____

_____

_____

_____

_____

_____

_____

_____

_____

_____

_____

_____

_____

REFERENCES

American Psychiatric Association. (2013). *Diagnostic and statistical manual of mental disorders (5th ed)*.

Baumrind, D. (1967). *Child care practices anteceding three patterns of preschool behavior. Genetic Psychology Monographs, 75(1), 43-88.*

Jones, Anna M.; Nadai, Alessandro S. De; Arnold, Elysse B.; McGuire, Joseph F.; Lewin, Adam B.; Murphy, Tanya K.; Storch, Eric A. (2013-02-01). "Psychometric Properties of the Obsessive Compulsive Inventory: Child Version in Children and Adolescents with Obsessive–Compulsive Disorder." Child Psychiatry & Human Development. 44 (1): 137–151. doi:10.1007/s10578-012-0315-0. ISSN 0009-398X. PMID 22711294.

Last, Cynthia G.; Strauss, Cyd C. (1989). "Obsessive—compulsive disorder in childhood." *Journal of Anxiety Disorders*. **3** (4): 295–302. doi:10.1016/0887-6185(89)90020-0.

Leckman, JF; Bloch, MH; King, RA (2009). "Symptom dimensions and subtypes of obsessive-compulsive disorder: a developmental perspective." Dialogues in Clinical Neuroscience. **11** (1): 21–33. PMC 3181902. PMID 19432385..

Ayres, A. Jean (1972). Sensory integration and learning disorders. Los Angeles: Western Psychological Services. ISBN 0-87424-303-3. OCLC 590960.

Ayres AJ (1972). "Types of sensory integrative dysfunction among disabled learners." *Am J Occup Ther.* 26 (1): 13–8. PMID 5008164.

CONCLUSION

I hope this book has encouraged you to seek a more balanced family life. More structure improves parent-child communication and builds the foundation for a stronger relationship with your child. It is my hope that you will use the tips and recommendations given to effectively manage the behavioral needs of your child and help them blossom. IT'S TIME FOR **YOUR** CHILD TO TRANSFORM FROM CHALLENGE TO CHAMPION.

THANK YOU

I would like to express my sincere gratitude to my great aunts and uncles, Mary and Walter Johnson, Simon and Georgia Gilmore, and Lorie Jones and Lurleen Roach for your love, prayers, and support. To all my friends who have witnessed and endured the hardships of my transformation, I say thank you for your encouragement. Thank you to all my extended family, friends, and supporters who have encouraged me throughout the years and have helped me achieve my dream of having a global impact.

I want to extend a special thank you to my business coach, Dr. Drai, my Medical Moguls family, my branding coach, Jai Stone, and my publishing company. Thank you to my mentors and professors from South Carolina State University, University of Louisville and Virginia Commonwealth University. Words can not express how much I appreciate you and may God continue to richly bless you all.

CONTACT US

Be sure to like and follow us on:

Facebook@DrMildredPeds

Twitter@DrMildredPeds

Instagram@DrMildredPeds

Pinterest@DrMildredPeds

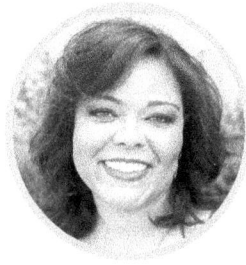

ABOUT THE AUTHOR

Dr. Mildred Carson is an author, speaker, consultant, and board-certified pediatrician with 15 years of clinical practice. She holds a Bachelor of Science in Biology from South Carolina State University and an MD from the University of Louisville School of Medicine. Dr. Carson is also a health coach, certified by the Institute for Integrative Nutrition. She is an active member of her community and has been recognized as an unsung hero for her excellence in the area of healthcare. In her years of experience and current role as medical director of a behavioral health agency, Dr. Carson has helped over 10,000 children and families. She is passionate about her vision for a world of happier, healthier children.

Dr. Carson is dedicated to building stronger families by helping parents to better discipline their children through more effective methods of communication.

Learn more at www.drmildredpeds.com

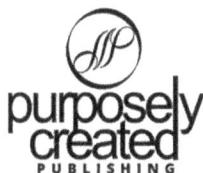

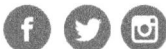